The BOObies

(And that nasty thing called Cancer)

Ceara Hayden

The Boobies

Published in 2018 by A Spark in the Sand
94 Beach St
Askam-in-Furness
Cumbria
LA16 7BH
England

www.asparkinthesand.co.uk

Copyright © Ceara Hayden 2018
ISBN 978-1-9998240-6-8

For my Mummy...

the strongest woman I know

In the UK...

1 in 8 women will be affected by Breast Cancer in their lifetime.

1,000 will die from it every month.

But... survival rates are increasing every day.

And this is due to better awareness, screening and treatment.

What follows is a story of optimism and survival.

Whilst this is not everyone's outcome, with your help - it can be.

So... Give your bOObies a hug. Check them. Feel them. Then tell others to do the same*.

*Their own, of course.

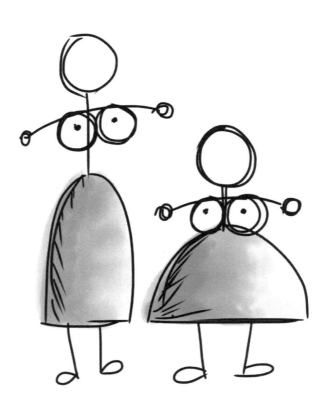

Some bOObies are big. Some bOObies are small.
Thin people, fat people, the short and the tall.
They all have these 'things' stuck to their chests,
Hidden under bras and beneath strappy vests.

They're handy for babies, supplying with milk,
And are weirdly seductive to men (when in silk).

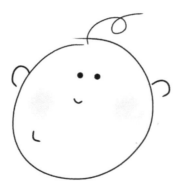

They're generally fine, causing no real issue,
Until something crops up underneath the breast tissue.

Sometimes, just because, and no one knows why,
Naughty cells turn quite horrid and then start to pry.
They gang up together and form a big lump,
Then hide behind tissue, a bra or a bump.

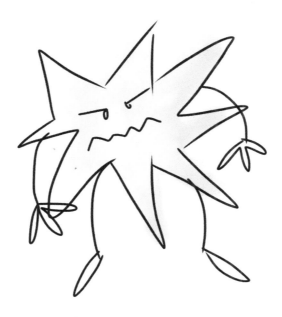

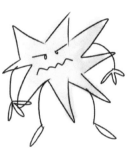

They can sit there in peace, growing in size,
And they think that they're clever and ever so wise.

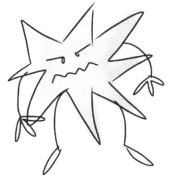

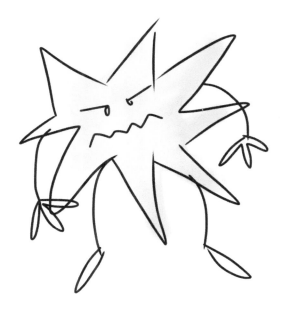

Then along comes the doctor with his special machine,
Seeking them out - ha - they think they're not seen!

The cells start to quiver - they're all of a wreck,
And out comes the lump, just like that - bloomin' heck.

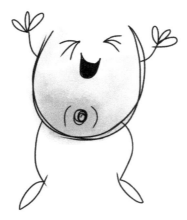

They're gone in a flash as the lump disappears,
As the boobies emit a loud, grateful cheer.

Alas, some stubborn cells can often remain,
They're the ones that are nuisances, a right real pain.
But fear not, they'll be zapped with the point of a beam,
And blitzed right away for being evil and mean.

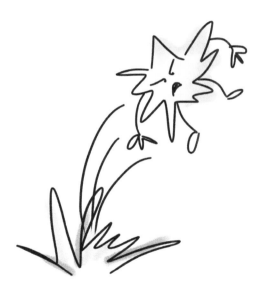

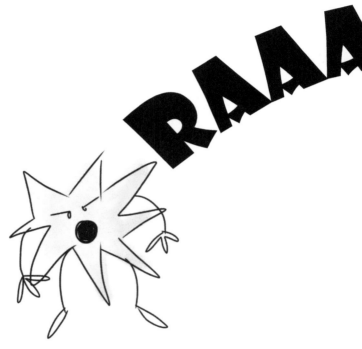

Sometimes that won't do for the the worst of the lot,
Who sit scheming and inventing plans to be plot.
They cause quite a mischief, they're sneaky they are,
Biding their time, then jumping out with a "raaaaarrr."

AARRR!

But they don't get a chance, as they're stopped in their tracks,
By a wondrous cure - a chemical "smack."
This cleaner - like Dettol - or bleach you could say,
Is ready to bash them and wipe them away.

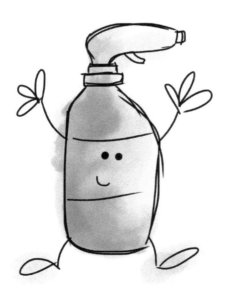

This powerful stuff is really quite strong,
Telling cells firmly that they are quite wrong.

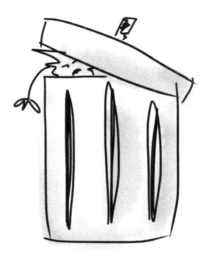

Then every few weeks, the cleaner comes in,
Mopping up all the cells to put in the bin.

Then after a while, there aren't many left there,
"It's just one more treatment," the bOObies declare!
Then they're sparkly clean, from the inside and out,
From where the mean, nasty cells can no longer sprout.

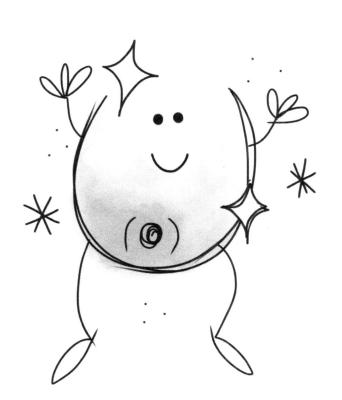

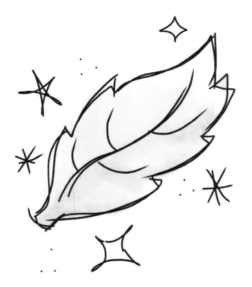

Once all that is over, there's a sigh of relief,
As the bOObies turn over a new, shiny leaf.
It's been quite a battle - the biggest of all,
But the bOObies fought hard in this very brawl.

- The End -

This book has been a labour of love. But it wouldn't have happened without the support and help of some amazingly, incredible people.

Firstly - to the Mother. For being an inspiration to us all.
Secondly, to Daddy Hayden - for being there for Mum when I couldn't be.
To Micaela - for looking after Mum from 'afar' (heaven is really rather far away).

Thanks to Amy, for all the help and tips on publishing my first book. I'm eternally grateful to Michael Southorn for the proofreading and James Clark for all the printing help. You legends.

And finally - big thanks to Chris... for telling me off when I became distracted.

(Oh... and of course, Oscar Bunny. For sitting on my first drafts).

Money raised from the sale of the book shall be sent to CoppaFeel!
An incredible charity on a mission to get people to boobie-check more, as one day it could save their life.

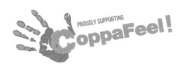

PROUDLY SUPPORTING CoppaFeel!